Clove Bud Essential Oil

Benefits, Properties, Applications, Studies & Recipes

by Ann Sullivan

Published in USA by:

Ann Sullivan
217 N. Seacrest Blvd #9
Boynton Beach
FL 33425

© Copyright 2017

ISBN-13: ISBN-13: 978-1546782278
ISBN-10: 1546782273

Table of Contents

Introduction

What are essential oils, and how might they be used for therapeutic purposes?

Essential oils are ultra-potent oils, extracted from plants and flowers that have been utilized in medicine for centuries. Presently, they're most commonly used to supplement pharmaceutical medication, but they can also be an effective alternative to pharmaceuticals if you don't have access to them. Before you dismiss essential oils to support the body's natural defenses against injuries and illness, look at the historical evidence of the oils' medicinal competence in practice. Your average age-old medical text will demonstrate that essential oils, herbs, and plenty of other natural ingredients have, for thousands of years, successfully enhanced immune function to meet and defeat any number of ailments and injuries. Though traditional medicine is considered "alternative" now, it was once the gold standard. And, frankly, perhaps it still should be, as these natural age-tested remedies can fortify the body's battlements against everything from simple maladies, like headaches, cuts and bruises, to serious diseases, like cancer.

Essential oils are deemed "essential," because the oils are composed of the "essence" of the plant. The difference between essential oils and other oils – like olive oil or vegetable oil, for instance – is that essential oils have high volatility and reduced fixation, which results in faster evaporation, enabling their popular use in aromatherapy.

Even at high temperatures, olive and vegetable oils don't evaporate.

Essential oils are especially necessary when it comes to a major natural or man-made disaster or some potential viral outbreak. In these types of dire situations, you may not have quick access (or any access at all) to your standard pharmaceutical supply; so, essential oils, along with other alternative therapies, will be your go-to wellness aids in the case of social collapse, viral outbreak or devastating natural disaster. When medical access is null and void, alternatives to our modern-day standard are the only chance we have to keep pathogens at bay.

You probably don't realize that you already use essential oils every day. They're in perfumes, shampoos, soaps, ointments...they're even used in furniture polish. Why are they found in so many aromatic products? Well, basically, because essential oils are super concentrated aromatic liquids, so their scent is remarkably strong. Let's put this into perspective: to steam tea, you use a few leaves of peppermint or juniper; to produce a single ounce of essential oil, five whole *pounds* of peppermint or juniper leaves are required. Some sources claim that to produce twelve pounds of essential oil would necessitate an acre of peppermint, juniper, or any other oil you're looking to produce en masse. Unlike vegetable oil, you don't often find concentrated therapeutic-grade essential oils sold by the tub load; instead the oils are often sold in easily carried small, dark bottles, perfect for your GOOD bag (Get Out of Dodge). Which is exactly what this book is aiming to help you do – get out of dodge with your most vital of essential oils intact, in particular a good supply of clove bud essential oil.

Why clove bud, you ask? Well, to get you quickly up to speed on this most essential of oils, below we've provided a condensed synopsis of clove bud, after which we'll outline in greater detail the oil's history, properties, and common therapeutic uses, so that you – the consumer – might have a better understanding of the oil's benefits and applications. We've even provided supportive remedies for pure clove, as well as blended recipes that incorporate the valuable oil. Chapter 3 will further detail past scientific research on clove bud essential oil.

Now, let's get down to it.

Essential Oil 101: The Basics of Clove Bud

Summary: Clove, or Eugenia caryophyllata, is as old as time, dating back to ancient India and China. This multi-purpose oil was traditionally used in Chinese medicine to support bronchitis, hernia and diarrhea. It has also been commonly used to combat digestive issues, intestinal parasites, toothaches and skin infections. Clove oil is anti-everything – anti-bacterial, anti-viral, anti-fungal; you name it, clove oil is likely to support the body's defenses against it.

When choosing your clove essential oil, it is important to know that there are hundreds of variations of the clove species and several specific chemotypes. As these different species have grown in different climates, the chemical properties of each chemotype are altered. Having different properties means that differing chemotypes of clove can be used for different applications.

Description: Clove oil is commonly extracted through steam distillation. The buds are most often used. The oil is golden brown or yellow in color, medium and oily in consistency, and has a strong warm spicy and woody scent.

Uses: Beyond those applications previously mentioned, additional uses for clove essential oil include supporting the body's natural function against pain, arthritis, cardiovascular disease, rheumatism, digestive issues, vomiting, nausea, diarrhea, viral infections, bacterial infections, fungal infections, flu, hepatitis, skin issues, parasites, ulcers, cataracts, inflammation, lice, wounds, insect bites/stings, poison oak, lupus, skin cancer, warts, acne, thyroid dysfunction, asthma, sprains, toothache, immune system deficiency, and addiction. When it comes to mood and emotion, clove oil can improve memory and concentration. It can also help combat depression and fatigue.

Properties: Antioxidant, antibacterial, anti-inflammatory, antifungal, antiparasitic, antiviral, analgesic, aphrodisiac, antiseptic, stimulant, digestive, and disinfectant.

Application: Dilute 1:4 with a carrier oil. You can apply topically, diffuse or use as a dietary supplement.

Safety Precautions: Clove has been approved by the FDA for internal consumption and so can be used as a dietary supplement. If you have sensitive skin, dilute heavily, as clove may irritate. Clove is also an anti-coagulant, so if you're using it alongside blood thinners, their effects will be enhanced. If you are an alcoholic, are hemophiliac, or have prostate cancer or liver or kidney issues, do not use clove oil.

Fun facts: Clove's names is derived from the Latin word for "nail" which is "clavus."

And the medicinal qualities of clove oil prove to be hard as nails. The Dutch conquered the Penang people of the Spice Islands in the sixteenth century, ridding the islands of all the clove trees in the process. Prior to this destruction, there had never been a health epidemic amongst the natives.

Another interesting fact about clove is that it helped protect against the 15th century plague. Thieves who stole from graves during the time combined the effective oil in their special recipe, called "Four Thieves Vinegar."

Chapter 1 – Benefits of Clove Bud Essential Oil

Clove bud essential oil offers several therapeutic benefits; but you may be wondering what these benefits are. In this chapter, we'll take a closer look at the history of clove bud and its many uses.

Cultivation of Clove Bud

Eugenia caryophyllata is a species of clove tree that produces the aromatic flower bud from which the essential oil is extracted. Clove trees are evergreens that can grow up to 12 meters tall, with big leaves and pale green flower buds that turn bright red when they're mature. The cloves are ripe for harvesting, when they reach around 2 cm long. Clove buds are commonly used as a spice and are native to Indonesia, though the trees are now commercially cultivated in India, Pakistan, Tanzania, Sri Lanka, Madagascar, and Zanzibar, as well.

A History of Clove Bud

The history of clove bud dates all the way back to the third century BCE, where it's said that the Chinese were required to chew clove buds before speaking with the leader of the Han Dynasty, in order that they address him with fresh breath. Cloves were also discovered in a Syrian vessel by archeologists, which dates to around 1721 BCE. The clove trade became particularly profitable during the Middle Ages, when Muslim sailors dealt with merchants along the Indian Ocean route. Cloves were such a popular commodity in those days that they even got a mention in the famous *Arabian Nights*, where the characters were oft trading in cloves from India.

Only recently have clove trees spread to other continents. In the beginning, they only grew on the Spice Islands, where the oldest clove tree in the world, clocking in at around 400 years old, still stands. Clove's rarity made it a hot commodity, so much so that in the 17th century, the Dutch East India Company attempted to monopolize its trade control over the spice. Though a limit on exportation of the spice was enforced, the trade could not be monopolized, as clove trees were more widely spread across the Moluccas than could be policed.

Now used in international cuisine across the globe, clove is an especially valued spice in Middle Eastern dishes, as well as in Africa and Asia, where they're used in curries, meat dishes, marinades, and fruit dishes. They're also combined with sugar and lemon and used to flavor hot beverages. Often accompanied by cinnamon and cumin, the strength of the buds' aroma is favored in Mexican cuisine, where it's frequently paired with basil, vanilla, allspice, red wine, anise, citrus peel, peppercorn, and even onion.

In its native home in Indonesia, clove has historically been smoked in cigarettes called kretek, which can also be found in the US, Asia, and Europe. Moreover, the strong scent of clove has enabled the spice to serve as an insect repellant, particularly for ants.

Chinese, Ayurvedic, and western medicine and dentistry have long used clove as a painkiller, especially when it comes to tooth pain, cavity, or dental decay. Clove has been a key ingredient in the making of toothpaste and, combined with zinc oxide, has been used for temporary cavity fillings.

Other traditional medical applications include stomach, kidney, and spleen support, especially in Chinese medicine where the warming ability of clove is said to fortify the kidney and help regulate the digestive tract. The spice has long been applied topically, aroma therapeutically, or ingested for digestive support. In Tibetan medicine, cloves are still used in medicinal teas, as well as in topical applications, including muscle balms for the oil's analgesic quality.

Chemical Components

To generate the essential oil from clove bud, the buds must be steam distilled. This results in the oil's key chemical components, which are primarily eugenol, benzene, ethanol, thymol, hexane, flavonoids, and methylene chloride.

Main Properties of Clove Bud Essential Oil

Along with the properties previously mentioned in the introduction, clove bud oil possesses antioxidant, antibacterial, anti-inflammatory, antifungal, antiparasitic, antiviral, analgesic, aphrodisiac, antiseptic, stimulant, digestive, and disinfectant properties. With such a versatile range, clove bud is well equipped to fight off any pathogen in the body's path.

Clove bud, as mentioned, is composed of eugenol, benzene, ethanol, thymol, hexane, flavonoids, and methylene chloride. These components are what instill the enormously beneficial properties within clove bud essential oil. We'll outline these properties below.

Antioxidant

Anything high in antioxidants – whether fruit, beans, or essential oils – is a powerful advocate for your body. Antioxidants both protect against free radicals and repair their damage. What are free radicals? Free radicals are destructive chemicals that invade your body, produced by substances both inside and out. Some free radicals (or oxidants) form through normal bodily reactions, like inflammation, metabolism and aerobic respiration. Other free radicals form outside the body, but enter it due to exposure. These include harmful pollutants, toxins, smoking, alcohol, X-rays, and UV rays, to name a few. Although our bodies produce their own antioxidants, these often become damaged as we grow older; thus, introducing antioxidants into our bodies allows these nutrients and enzymes to assist in chemical reactions which destroy the oxidants or free radicals. Clove bud essential oil is a moderate antioxidant, aiming to detox the body of free radicals that lead to disease.

Antibacterial

Clove bud's antibacterial properties make it a powerful protectant against diseases produced by bacteria, such as oral, digestive and urinary tract bacterial infection. What's great is that, unlike some prescription drugs, clove bud has no ill effects on bodily wellness or on the healthy natural flora that exists within the stomach and intestines.

Anti-inflammatory

External or internal inflammation can be reduced using clove bud essential oil. For instance, if you or your patient has swollen fingers from arthritis or a swollen knee from a sport's injury, oral application of clove bud essential oil may decrease irritation or redness, while also soothing the pain that accompanies inflammation.

Antifungal

While bacteria and viruses are plenty evil, fungi commonly lead to the deadliest infections, whether external or internal. Your ears, throat and nose are the most likely to become infected by fungi, the infections of which can be both excruciating and unsightly. If left untreated, fungal infections can kill, as they may spread to the brain. Clove bud essential oil protects against these infections and more and is particularly effective against skin infections.

Antiparasitic

Parasites include such mites as fleas, bedbugs, tapeworms, mosquitoes, and lice – pretty much any irritating insect, internal or external, which feeds off the body in one way or another. The human body is a tasty meal to parasites, which can sometimes lead to the transmission of communicable diseases through their feasting off various meals. Clove bud essential oil is the answer. Its antiparasitic properties will combat mosquitoes, fleas, bedbugs and lice when applied topically, and intestinal worms when taken orally.

Antiviral

The antiviral protection that clove bud essential oil grants will essentially enhance the immune system, building up a tougher wall of security that most colds, measles or mumps are unlikely to scale. By boosting white blood cell count and function, this immune stimulant will ensure that your body is better prepared to protect against deadly viral infections.

Analgesic

As an analgesic, clove bud essential oil supports pain relief, acting on the central nervous system to fortify the body's natural defenses against inflammation and supporting relief from pain receptor sensation. dysmenorrhea.

Aphrodisiac

As an aphrodisiac, clove bud can help stimulate sexual arousal, thereby overriding impotence, frigidity, low libido, and erectile dysfunction.

Antiseptic

The antiseptic and disinfectant properties of clove bud essential oil can be reaped topically, applied directly to wounds, or even through burning; the smoke from the oil may help destroy airborne germs. Internal use will help keep the wounds from becoming infections, while external use will support the body's natural function in inhibiting tetanus.

Stimulant

Stimulants are often referred to as "uppers." This is because they produce mental or physical improvements or temporary enhancements of your bodily functions. For instance, you may grow more alert and awake or quicker on your feet after using a stimulant. Clove bud essential oil can provide this temporary boost in mental and physical function, especially when it comes to the immune system.

Digestive

By boosting the production of absorptive enzymes, the digestibility of nutrients, and the secretion of digestive juices, clove bud essential oil aids the digestive tract significantly, which can make a significant impact on your overall wellness by increasing those nutrients you absorb from food.

Disinfectant

As a disinfectant, clove bud can be added to household cleaners to disinfect your home. The oil eliminates contamination, which means your household will be healthier, overall, and will fall sick less often. Clove bud can be used purely or blended with other oils to clean dishes, clothing, and practically any surface.

Common Medicinal Uses

Traditionally used to enhance the body's defenses against infections and diseases, clove bud essential oil remains a significant immune system stimulant, protecting against several conditions, whether viral, fungal, or bacterial. Clove bud supports overall wellness and organ function, while mentally uplifting and improving concentration. Let's take a closer look at the common uses for this oil.

Immune System Booster

Clove bud is a superb immune system support which boosts circulation and increases white blood cell count. The oil's chemical components deliver incredible antifungal, antibacterial, and antiviral properties, making it akin to an immune shield braced to fight off angry bacterial strains, like salmonella, E. coli and staph infections. With such strong armor, this immune stimulant will ensure that your body is better prepared to protect against deadly infections.

Skin Care

Clove bud oil supports the body's defenses against acne, wrinkles, dryness, and other skin issues. The oil's properties invigorate dull skin, while cleansing and eliminating excess oil. Whether using clove bud essential oil to defy skin aging or to reduce adolescent skin issues, like pimples and acne, the antiseptic, disinfectant, and anti-inflammatory properties are superb for skin issues, bar none.

Stress Disorders

Whether it be physical stress or mental stress, clove bud's aroma, in conjunction with its therapeutic properties, enable its use in the support of stress disorders, like upset nerves, anxiety, melancholy, and depression. It can help soothe mental fatigue and refresh cognitive function. The oil induces restful sleep, stimulates concentration, and strengthens overall mental wellbeing.

Headache & Nausea

One of clove bud's simplest but most effective medicinal uses is to relieve headache pain and nausea. With a simple rub of the diluted oil on the temples and forehead, the calming, soothing properties of clove bud quickly eliminate the strongest and most stubborn of headaches, as both the refreshing scent and the oil's anti-inflammatory and analgesic properties help to alleviate tension. You can also simply inhale the scent from the bottle to soothe both headaches and nausea from motion sickness.

Respiratory Issues

As an anti-inflammatory, clove bud essential oil calms coughing by opening the airways. Bronchitis, congestion, asthma, sinusitis, cough, and other respiratory issues can be supported with clove bud essential oil, as the oil promotes a healthy respiratory tract, soothes the throat, and clears nasal passages.

Digestion

As a digestive aid, clove bud essential oil's collective properties stimulate digestive enzyme secretion which serves to support issues like constipation, upset stomach, flatulence, indigestion, heartburn, and stomach cramps. Eugenol, one of clove bud's main chemical components, is largely responsible for these effects. As clove is often used as a spice, particularly in Indian dishes, the digestive properties are coupled with an enrichment of culinary flavor.

Blood Circulation

Clove bud oil's coolant effect produces major responses in the body, among them, increased blood circulation. When the oil vapor touches the olfactory nerve ends, the pulse quickens and blood circulates, providing more oxygen to the body's organs and, especially, to the brain, which promotes cognitive function. The oxygenation to the brain also serves to protect against dementia, Alzheimer's and other neural degenerative diseases. Moreover, the oil reduces body temperature and boosts the metabolism.

Diabetes & Blood Sugar

Several studies have been done on clove bud's

relationship to insulin and, thereby, its potential application to diabetic wellness. What these studies have found is that clove bud essential oil helps regulate the production of insulin in the pancreas, which aids diabetic management by maintaining blood sugar levels. Maintaining a steady blood sugar level and reducing the dangerous drops or spikes that those suffering from diabetes are occasion to is also supported by the oil's blood circulating properties and its ability to stimulate proper metabolic function.

Bone Health

Clove bud is rich in phenolic compounds and those compound derivatives; these include its primary component, eugenol, and flavonoids, flavones, and isoflavones. These components support bone durability and density, making the oil an effective source when it comes to strengthening bone health. Clove bud can help decelerate the aging process of bones, combatting osteoporosis and other degenerative bone conditions.

Safety Precautions & Common Applications

Safety

Certain adverse effects may evolve when using pure essential oils. Some essential oils should not be used when pregnant, for example, as they may cause miscarriage. Allergic reactions, too, may occur, especially when applied topically. Always administer an allergy test before committing fully to topical application. When used with other medications, essential oils may react negatively. If you are on any current prescription medications or have a chronic illness, such as high blood pressure, epilepsy or liver disease, then researching the effects of essential oils against your own personal medical history will eliminate any potentially problematic issues.

Clove bud has been approved by the FDA for internal consumption and so can be used as a dietary supplement. Clove is also an anti-coagulant, so if you're using it alongside blood thinners, their effects will be enhanced. If you are an alcoholic, are hemophiliac, or have prostate cancer or liver or kidney issues, do not use clove oil. If you have sensitive skin, dilute heavily and test before extensive use. Otherwise, dilute 1:4 with a carrier oil. You can apply topically, diffuse or use as a dietary supplement.

Blends

Oftentimes, essential oils are manufactured as blends of several pure oils. For instance, the Protective Blend of certain brands is a mix of cinnamon, clove, rosemary, and eucalyptus. This blend can be used to boost the immune system to help support colds, viruses and flus. The downside to blends is that the more oils added to the mix, the higher the probability your patient may react negatively to the blend if he/she is prone to allergies. There is also the possibility of phototoxicity when working with blends, particularly if they include citrus oils. Be sure to read your labels before administering.

Regardless of these possible effects, essential oils are a viable option for supporting several conditions. Those looking to support or maintain their own personal wellness, or that of their families', should become educated on the uses of essential oils, their natural remedies and the methods of application. Only then can you begin building your kit of essential oils for survival.

Chapter 2 – Recipes for Clove Bud Essential Oil

In this chapter, we'll offer various recipes for clove bud essential oil, both for pure clove bud applications and blends. For pure applications, we've provided the appropriate dosage and method of administration to support specific ailments, from addiction to viral infections. When it comes to blends, herbalists and aromatherapists often combine clove bud essential oil with basil, cinnamon, rose, rosemary, grapefruit, orange, lemon, lavender, peppermint, nutmeg, and geranium. We'll offer some fantastic blending options in the second half of this chapter.

Pure Applications

Addiction

To help combat addiction, dilute clove essential oil in a 1:4 ratio with a carrier oil and apply topically, massaging over the solar plexus and the heart. You can also place a drop of oil on the tip of the tongue and take internally, or administer aromatically, diffusing throughout the home or inhaling directly from the bottle.

Athlete's Foot

Relieve athlete's foot by diluting clove essential oil in a 1:4 ratio with a carrier oil and massaging the solution into your feet. You can also add two drops of clove to a foot bath or soak a pair of socks in warm water with two drops of clove and wear them for a half hour. Place one drop in shoes to rid of contact fungus and for extended support.

Blood Clots

To support the body's natural defenses against blood clots, topically apply clove bud essential oil, diluted in a 1:4 ratio with a carrier oil, over the area of concern. You can also diffuse or take internally by adding a drop to a glass of water. *Ask your doctor to support this application before use.

Candida

Eliminate candida by diluting clove bud essential oil in a 1:4 ratio with a carrier oil and massaging over affected area, into the soles of the feet, and over the abdomen. You can also take clove orally, through use in a capsule or as a food additive.

Cataracts

To support the body's defenses against cataracts, dilute 1-2 drops of clove essential oil in a 1:4 ratio with a carrier oil and apply topically, massaging into the toes and the reflex points of the feet.

Codependency

If you're feeling intense codependency, clove may help break from this mindset. To administer, diffuse throughout the room or inhale directly.

Control Issues

Whether you find yourself lacking self-control or attempting to dominate others, you may administer clove bud essential oil to stimulate or reign in control issues. Apply topically, after diluting it in a 1:4 ratio with a carrier oil. Massage it into the soles of the feet. You can also diffuse throughout the room to support this issue.

Corns

Eliminate corns by diluting 1-2 drops of clove essential oil in a 1:4 ratio with a carrier oil and applying topically to the affected area up to three times daily.

Courage

To enhance courage or bravery, place a drop of clove

essential oil into your hands, rub your palms together, cup them over your nose, and breathe deeply in and out for several minutes. Use daily for the best results.

Diarrhea

If you're experiencing diarrhea, clove bud essential oil is the answer. Apply topically by diluting the oil in a 1:4 ratio with a carrier oil and massaging it into the abdomen in a counterclockwise motion, or place a drop of the oil in your drinking water throughout the day.

Digestive Aid

Clove bud aids the digestive tract and can be taken orally or topically. Place a drop into your drinking water for internal administration or dilute the oil in a 1:4 ratio with a carrier oil and apply topically to the abdomen in a clockwise motion and into the reflex points of the feet. You can also diffuse throughout the home.

Disinfectant

Clove bud is a fantastic ingredient to use in homemade cleaning products, as the oil's antibacterial and antiviral properties make it a superb disinfectant. Add a few drops to your commercial cleaning product or, better yet, make your own! Diffusing throughout your home will also improve the air quality.

Empowerment

Feel empowered by placing a drop of clove essential oil into your hands, rubbing your palms together, cupping them over your nose, and breathing deeply in and out for several minutes. Use daily for the best results. You can also diffuse throughout your home to empower others.

Fear

To help eliminate unwarranted fear, dilute clove bud essential oil in a 1:4 ratio with a carrier oil and apply topically, massaging over the solar plexus and the heart. You can also administer aromatically, diffusing throughout the home or inhaling directly from the bottle.

Fever

Clove bud supports the body's natural defenses against fever in that it helps regulate body temperature while, at the same time, fighting off infection. Diffuse throughout the home or place a drop in a glass of drinking water and take internally.

Flatulence

Relieve gas by diluting clove bud essential oil in a 1:4 ratio with a carrier oil and massaging into the abdomen in a clockwise motion. You can also place a drop in a glass of water and take orally.

Fungal Infections

Depending on the type of fungal infection, combat it through internal, topical, or aromatic application, according to its location. For instance, if you have athlete's foot, topical application may be the easiest and most direct solution. If you have an internal fungal infection, oral application would be more appropriate.

Healing

Accelerate the healing process by applying 1-2 drops of clove bud essential oil, diluted in a 1:4 ratio with a carrier oil, over the affected area.

Viral Hepatitis

Support the body's natural defenses against viral hepatitis by diffusing or steaming two drops of clove bud essential oil in a pan of water. Remove the steaming pan from the stove, pour into a bowl, place a towel over your head and inhale. If you don't feel it's done its job the first time, you can reheat that same water and use it once more without adding more oil. You can also dilute clove bud in a 1:4 ratio with a carrier oil and apply topically, massaging over the liver and into the soles of the feet every day.

Herpes Complex

Combat herpes complex virus by diluting clove bud essential oil in a 1:4 ratio with a carrier oil and applying topically, massaging it into the soles of the feet, alternating between right and left each day.

Hodgkin's Disease

Support the symptoms of Hodgkin's Disease diluting clove bud essential oil in a 1:4 ratio with a carrier oil and applying topically, massaging it over the affected area daily.

Hormonal Balance

Support hormonal balance by diluting clove bud essential oil in a 1:4 ratio with a carrier oil and massaging into the reflex points of the feet daily.

Hypothyroidism

Support healthy thyroid function by diffusing clove bud essential oil. You can also administer topically by diluting the oil in a 1:4 ratio with a carrier oil and applying over the thyroid every day.

Infection

To fight off infection, dilute clove bud essential oil in a 1:4 ratio with a carrier oil and apply topically to the affected area or to the soles of the feet up to three times daily. You can also diffuse throughout the room; whichever application is more appropriate to your specific infection.

Insecticide

To rid of bus throughout the home, apply 1 drop of clove bud essential oil to a cotton ball and place near problem areas, like entryways, cupboards, closets, etc. For a similar effect, you can diffuse the oil throughout the room.

Intestinal Parasites

Rid of intestinal parasites by diluting clove bud essential oil in a 1:4 ratio with a carrier oil and massaging it into the abdomen and the soles of the feet. You can also add a drop to your drinking water.

Liver Support

Support liver function by diluting clove bud essential oil in a 1:4 ratio with a carrier oil; then apply topically, massaging over the affected area and into the reflex points of the feet. You can also place a drop in your drinking water and take internally daily.

Lupus

Combat lupus by adding a couple drops of clove essential oil to a veggie capsule or your drinking water and taking internally. You can also apply topically, diluting the oil in a 1:4 ratio with a carrier oil and massaging it over the affected area and into the reflex points of the feet.

Macular Degeneration

Clove bud's regenerative quality makes it an effective support to the nervous system. Dilute clove bud essential oil in a 1:4 ratio with a carrier oil and apply topically over the affected area or massage into the reflex points of the feet. You may also diffuse the oil throughout the home.

Memory

Stimulate the memory by steaming two drops of clove bud essential oil in a pan of water. Then remove the steaming pan from the stove, pour into a bowl, place a towel over your head and inhale. If you don't feel it's done its job the first time, you can reheat that same water and use it once more without adding more oil. You can also diffuse the oil wherever you study or work. Additionally, try inhaling directly, add a few drops to bathwater, or dilute in a

1:4 ratio with a carrier oil and massage into the base of the toes or the back of the neck.

Metabolism Balance

Maintain a balanced metabolism by adding a couple drops of clove essential oil to a veggie capsule or your drinking water and taking internally. You can also diffuse throughout the room to support this issue.

Mold

Mold, mildew and fungus can cause a slew of wellness problems. Clove bud essential oil will help rid of these fungi throughout your home. Apply a few drops directly to the affected area, diffuse, or place a few drops in your cleaning products.

Muscle Pain

To relieve muscle pain or body aches, dilute clove bud essential oil in a 1:4 ratio with a carrier oil and massage the solution into the affected area, toward the heart.

Osteoporosis

To alleviate the inflammation and pain of osteoporosis, dilute clove bud essential oil in a 1:4 ratio with a carrier oil and massage the solution into the affected area.

Plague

Protect against and help relieve symptoms of the plague by diluting clove bud essential oil with a carrier oil and massaging into the soles of the feet. You may also combat infection by diffusing throughout the home.

Poison Ivy/Oak

Relieve poison ivy or poison oak with a topical application of clove bud essential oil. Dilute in a 1:4 ratio and apply to the affected area to protect against infection, numb the sting, and accelerate healing.

Rheumatoid Arthritis

To combat the pain and inflammation of rheumatoid arthritis, dilute clove bud essential oil in a 1:4 ratio with a carrier oil and apply topically, massaging the oil into the joints. You can also simply diffuse or use the steam method. Steam two drops of the oil in a pan of water, remove the steaming pan from the stove, pour into a bowl, place a towel over your head and inhale. If you don't feel it's done its job the first time, you can reheat that same water and use it once more without adding more oil.

Ringworm

Ringworm can be targeted topically by diluting clove bud essential oil in a 1:4 ratio with a carrier oil and massaging over the affected area up to three times daily. Once the ringworm is eliminated, continue the application for 3-5 days following recovery.

Skin Cancer

To help protect against skin cancer or support its symptoms, dilute clove bud essential oil in a 1:4 ratio with a carrier oil and apply topically to affected area twice daily.

Sores (Skin or Oral)

Accelerate the healing of skin sores or oral sores (canker or cold) by diluting clove bud essential oil with a carrier oil and applying to the affected area twice daily.

Termites

Eliminate termites by adding a single drop of clove bud essential oil to a cotton ball and placing in the contaminated area. You can also diffuse throughout the room to enhance the aroma's effect.

Thyroid Dysfunction

Support healthy thyroid function by diffusing clove bud essential oil. You can also administer topically by diluting the oil in a 1:4 ratio with a carrier oil and applying over the thyroid every day.

Toothache

To help alleviate toothache, dilute 1 drop of clove bud essential oil with 1 teaspoon coconut oil and apply topically to the affected area.

Teething Pain

For teething pain in little ones, dilute 1 drop of clove bud essential oil in 1 tablespoon of coconut oil and apply directly to the affected area or dip a washcloth in a watered-down clove bud solution, freeze the washcloth, and allow the toddler to use as a chew toy.

Tumor (Lipoma)

Relieve tumors by diluting 1-2 drops of clove bud essential oil in a 1:4 ratio with a carrier oil and applying topically to the affected area twice daily.

Ulcer (Leg)

Target ulcers internally by placing a drop in each meal or glass of water, or externally by diluting clove bud essential oil in a 1:4 ratio with a carrier oil and applying topically, massaging into the stomach and into the reflex points of the feet.

Viral Infection

Nearly any infection can be subdued with clove bud essential oil. Dilute the essential oil in a 1:4 ratio with a carrier oil and apply topically, massaging over the affected area and into the soles of the feet up to three times daily.

Warts

To eliminate warts, dilute clove bud essential oil in a 1:4 ratio with a carrier oil and apply directly to the wart twice daily. Continue this application until the wart is removed.

Wounds

Enhance wound healing by adding a few drops of clove bud essential oil to a spray bottle filled with distilled water. Spray over the wound. You may also apply a few drops to a spritz bath and soak wound for 10-15 minutes. Lastly, you can dilute clove bud in a 1:4 ratio with a carrier oil and apply topically, massing into the affected area or the soles of the feet.

Blends

Aphrodisiac Massage Blend

Ingredients

- 1 drop Ginger Essential Oil
- 1 drop Clove Essential Oil
- 2 drops Cinnamon Essential Oil
- 2 drops Peppermint Essential Oil
- 3 drops Jasmine Essential Oil
- 3 drops Vanilla Absolute
- 2 ounces Carrier Oil

Directions

To stimulate sexual arousal for men and women, combine all ingredients in a small bowl, blending well. Apply in a full body massage or into the reflex points (*caution: cinnamon essential oil is hot and may irritate sensitive skin; if you are prone to skin irritation, increase the amount of carrier oil).

Aphrodisiac Scent

Ingredients

- 1 drop Clove Essential Oil
- 1 drop Cassia Essential Oil
- 3 drops Wild Orange Essential Oil
- 1 tsp Carrier Oil

Directions

In a small bowl or container, mix all ingredients until well combined. Apply to the pulse points for an attractive scent.

Arthritis

Ingredients

- 3 drops Oregano Essential Oil
- 3 drops Clove Essential Oil
- 1 tsp Carrier Oil

Directions

Relieve arthritic pain by combining all ingredients in a small glass container and applying topically, massaging into the affected area and the reflex points of the feet twice a day.

Bed Bug Remover

Ingredients

- 10 drops Eucalyptus Essential Oil
- 10 drops Rosemary Essential Oil
- 10 drops Lavender Essential Oil
- 3 drops Clove Essential Oil
- 1 tsp Vodka
- 1 cup Distilled Water

Directions

Get rid of bed bugs by combining all ingredients in a spritz bottle and shaking well. Spray over your sheets and mattress. Use as needed, shaking well before each use.

Colds

Ingredients

- 5 drops Oregano Essential Oil
- 5 drops Thyme Essential Oil
- 8 drops Clove Essential Oil

Directions

To stave off colds or relieve cold symptoms, place all ingredients into a "00" capsule, and ingest 1 capsule twice a day.

Cirrhosis of the Liver

Ingredients

- 2 drops Grapefruit Essential Oil
- 2 drops Clove Essential Oil
- 1 drop Geranium Essential Oil
- 1 drop Rosemary Essential Oil
- 1 tsp Carrier Oil

Directions

To support the liver and combat cirrhosis, combine all ingredients and apply topically over the region of the liver twice daily.

Diabetes

Ingredients

- 8 drops Cinnamon Essential Oil
- 8 drops Clove Essential Oil
- 10 drops Thyme Essential Oil
- 15 drops Rosemary Essential Oil
- 2 ounces V-6

Directions

To help maintain insulin levels, combine all ingredients and apply topically to feet and over pancreas.

Flu Virus

Ingredients

- 2 drops Clove Essential Oil
- 2 drops Lemon Essential Oil
- 3 drops Frankincense Essential Oil
- 8 drops Oregano Essential Oil

Directions

To support the body's natural defenses against the flu, place all ingredients into a "00" capsule, and ingest 1 capsule twice a day.

Four Thieves Oil

Ingredients

- 10 drops Rosemary Essential Oil
- 15 drops Eucalyptus Essential Oil
- 20 drops Cinnamon Bark Essential Oil
- 35 drops Lemon Essential Oil
- 40 drops Clove Bud Essential Oil
- 12 ounces Distilled Water

Directions

Combine all ingredients in a dark colored glass spray bottle and, during cold and flu season or if there's illness in the house, spray in all rooms to stimulate the immune system.

Hand Sanitizer

Ingredients

- 10 drops Clove Essential Oil
- 10 drops Cinnamon Essential Oil
- 10 drops Lemon Essential Oil
- 10 drops Eucalyptus Essential Oil
- 10 drops Rosemary Essential Oil
- 1 tsp Aloe Vera
- 3 ounces Distilled Water

Directions

Make a hand-sanitizing spray by combining all ingredients in a 4-ounce spray bottle. Shake well and use as needed, misting onto the hands and rubbing in until the solution evaporates. Shake before each use.

Headache Relief

Ingredients

- 5 drops Clove Essential Oil
- 6 drops Ginger Essential Oil
- 9 drops Peppermint Essential Oil
- 9 drops Wintergreen Essential Oil
- 4 tsps. Carrier Oil

Directions

To relieve headaches, combine all ingredients in a small bowl, blending well. Apply to the temples, forehead, back of the neck, the reflex points, or in a full body massage.

Immune-Boosting Topical Blend

Ingredients

- 5 drops Rosemary Essential Oil
- 8 drops Eucalyptus Essential Oil
- 10 drops Cinnamon Bark Essential Oil
- 18 drops Lemon Essential Oil
- 20 drops Clove Essential Oil

Directions

Combine all ingredients in a dark colored bottle and, during cold and flu season or if there's illness in the house, apply topically with a carrier oil to stimulate the immune system.

Intestinal Issues

Ingredients

- 1 drop Clove Essential Oil
- 1 drop Peppermint Essential Oil
- 1 drop Chamomile Essential Oil
- 2 drops Rosemary Essential Oil
- 5 mL Carrier Oil

Directions

To relieve intestinal issues, place all ingredients into a small bowl or container and blend thoroughly. Apply topically, massaging over the stomach.

Joyful & Uplifting Scent

Ingredients

- 3 drops Rosemary Essential Oil
- 4 drops Clove Essential Oil
- 6 drops Lemon Essential Oil
- 2 tsps. Vanilla Extract
- 1 ½ cups Water

Directions

Fill your home with a joyful and uplifting scent by mixing all ingredients in your crockpot until well combined. Simmer and allow the aroma to lift your spirit.

Prostate Supportive Blend

Ingredients

- 2 drops Frankincense Essential Oil
- 2 drops Invigorating Blend Essential Oil
- 1 drops Clove Essential Oil
- 1 drops Thyme Essential Oil
- 1 drops Lavender Essential Oil
- 1 tsp Carrier Oil

Directions

In a small bowl or container, mix all ingredients until well combined. Massage into the area below the genitals twice daily. You can also take the blend internally in a 00 capsule for up to six weeks, modified (double the recipe).

Room Disinfectant

Ingredients

- 6 drops Cinnamon Bark Essential Oil
- 6 drops Pine Essential Oil
- 5 drops Juniper Berry Essential Oil
- 3 drops Clove Essential Oil

Directions

In a glass, marble, porcelain or ceramic aroma lamp, combine the essential oils with water. Diffuse the oils and deeply breathe in the vapors.

Thyroid Support

Ingredients

- 10 drops Myrrh Essential Oil
- 12 drops Clove Essential Oil
- 12 drops Lemongrass Essential Oil
- 12 drops Peppermint Essential Oil
- 1 Tbsp. Coconut Oil

Directions

To support the thyroid, especially conditions like hypothyroidism, combine ingredients in a small glass bowl or jar, blending well. Apply topically, massaging over the thyroid daily.

Tooth Decay

Ingredients

- 20 drops Clove Essential Oil
- 20 drops Trace Minerals (or Calcium Powder)
- 4 Tbsps. Coconut Oil
- 2 Tbsps. Baking Soda
- 1 Tbsp. Xylitol (or 1/8 tsp Stevia)

Directions

To reverse cavities and combat tooth decay, combine all ingredients and use as a toothpaste.

Chapter 3 – Clove Bud Essential Oil Studies

Many studies have been done on essential oils to uncover and prove their therapeutic qualities. In the case of the great number of clove bud studies, many of the properties attributed to the essential oil (noted in this book and elsewhere) are quite often validated through the research from accredited universities and published by reputable scientific journals. In this chapter, we'll discuss a small portion of these studies. It's important to note that research on essential oils is constantly evolving. Keep up with any recent research, as it may turn up even further valuable uses for these miracle oils.

Study 1 – Antimicrobial Activity

In this study published by the *Brazilian Journal of Microbiology*, the antimicrobial activities of clove bud essential oil were examined, with the following results: "The influence of clove essential oil concentration, temperature and organic matter, in the antimicrobial activity of clove essential oil, was studied in this paper, through the determination of bacterial death kinetics. Escherichia coli, Staphylococcus aureus and Pseudomonas aeruginosa were the microorganisms selected for a biological test... (Results indicated that) Clove essential oil can be considered as a potential antimicrobial agent for external use."

This study tested the antibacterial activity against three bacteria: Escherichia coli, Staphylococcus aureus, and Pseudomonas aeruginosa. Escherichia coli is a Gram-negative bacterium that often causes serious food poisoning. Although the Gram-positive bacterium, Staphylococcus aureus, is part of the normal human skin flora and respiratory tract and is not typically pathogenic, those with compromised immune systems can potentially develop an infection from the bacteria. When this happens, S. aureus produces respiratory issues like sinusitis, skin infections, and even food poisoning. Pseudomonas aeruginosa is a common bacteria found in water, soil, skin flora, and in man-made environments. The bacteria thrives on moist surfaces, and so can threaten the hospital environment by finding its home on medical equipment, like catheters, which may result in cross-infection. It is, for instance, the bacterium which causes hot-tub rash. P. aeruginosa also attacks immunocompromised patients, infecting the urinary tract, airway, wounds, burns, and resulting in blood infections.

Clove essential oil showed high inhibition against these strains of bacteria and, thereby, could be used as a valuable antimicrobial agent for topical applications.

Reference
http://www.ncbi.nlm.nih.gov/pubmed/24031950

http://www.ncbi.nlm.nih.gov/pmc/articles/PMC3769004/pdf/bjm-43-1255.pdf

Study 2 – Menstruation (Dysmenorrhea)

In this study published by *Evidence-Based Complementary and Alternative Medicine*, the effects of clove bud essential oil on menstruation were examined, with the following results: "Dysmenorrhea is a common cause of sickness absenteeism from both classes and work. This study investigated the effect of aromatherapy massage on a group of nursing students who are suffering of primary dysmenorrhea... using the essential oils (cinnamon, clove, rose, and lavender in a base of almond oil)...During both treatment phases, the level and duration of menstrual pain and the amount of menstrual bleeding were significantly lower in the aromatherapy group than in the placebo group. These results suggests that aromatherapy is effective in alleviating menstrual pain, its duration and excessive menstrual bleeding. Aromatherapy can be provided as a nonpharmacological pain relief measure and as a part of nursing care given to girls suffering of dysmenorrhea, or excessive menstrual bleeding."

This study demonstrated the effectivity of clove essential oil against excessive menstrual bleeding and pain, a condition known as dysmenorrhea. After massaging the essential oil into the abdominal area during menses, both the amount of bleeding and pain were significantly reduced.

Reference

http://www.ncbi.nlm.nih.gov/pubmed/23662151

http://www.ncbi.nlm.nih.gov/pmc/articles/PMC3638625/pdf/ECAM2013-742421.pdf

Study 3 – Antibacterial Properties

In this study, available on PubMed, the antibacterial effects of clove essential oil on oral wellness were examined, with the following results: "To study the antibacterial activity of nine commercially available essential oils against Streptococcus mutans in vitro and to compare the antibacterial activity between each material...Cinnamon oil, lemongrass oil, cedarwood oil, clove oil and eucalyptus oil exhibit antibacterial property against S. mutans."

Streptococcus mutans is an oral bacteria which causes

cavities and tooth decay. Clove bud was among nine essential oils tested against this strain of bacteria and was found to be one of the most powerful in inhibiting S.mutans. This validates clove bud's use in oral health and suggests that the oil has potential in controlling oral infection-producing yeasts and bacteria.

Reference
http://www.ncbi.nlm.nih.gov/pubmed/22430697

Study 4 – Antioxidant & Antimicrobial Properties

In this study published in the *Journal of Oleo Science*, the antioxidant and antimicrobial properties of clove bud essential oil were examined, with the following results: "Clove bud essential oil (CEO) and its major individual phenolic constituent eugenol were formulated as nanoparticles in water-based microemulsion systems…The results of this study could have potential applications in water-based disinfectants, preservation and flavoring of food and in personal hygiene products. It may also have promising applications in the nutraceutical and functional beverage field."

This study was a comparative analysis of clove bud essential oil's activities when placed in a water-based micro-emulsion. The objective of this study was to see if the oil's main components were affected by the emulsion, in the event that clove may be used in water-based products. Clove bud essential oil and its major component, eugenol, were both shown to retain their antioxidant and antimicrobial properties in microemulsion, indicating their efficacy for potential use in personal hygiene products, food flavors and preservatives, disinfectants, and nutraceutical beverages.

Reference

http://www.ncbi.nlm.nih.gov/pubmed/23138253

https://www.jstage.jst.go.jp/article/jos/61/11/61_641/_pdf]

Study 5 – Foodborne Pathogens

In this study published in the *Journal of Agriculture & Food Chemistry*, the effects of clove bud essential oil on foodborne pathogens were examined, with the following results: "Meats need to be heated to inactivate foodborne pathogens such as Escherichia coli O157:H7. High-temperature treatment used to prepare well-done meats increases the formation of carcinogenic heterocyclic amines (HCAs). We evaluated the ability of plant extracts, spices, and essential oils to simultaneously inactivate E. coli O157:H7 and suppress HCA formation in heated hamburger patties…The results suggest that edible natural plant compounds have the potential to prevent foodborne infections as well as carcinogenesis in humans consuming heat-processed meat products."

A number of extracts, spices, and essential oils were tested against E.coli in ground beef, in order to determine their efficacy in combatting bacteria. E.coli, as stated in the first study of this chapter, is a Gram-negative bacterium that often causes serious food poisoning. A 1% clove bud oil application reduced the pathogen by 1.6 log CFU/g. These results indicate that clove bud essential oil, and other natural plant compounds, can help protect against foodborne infections caused by this bacteria.

Reference
http://www.ncbi.nlm.nih.gov/pubmed/22397498]

Study 6 – Antioxidant Activity

In this study published by *Scientia Pharmaceutica*, the antioxidant activity of clove bud essential oil were examined, with the following results: "The essential oil (EO) of clove bud dried fruits from Eugenia caryophyllus was obtained… To evaluate the possible antioxidant capacity of eugenol compounds including the clove bud EO…It was found that the prepared eugenol derivatives had a more potent free radical scavenger activity than the reference compounds."

This study evaluates the antioxidant activity of clove bud essential oil. Antioxidants protect against free radicals and repair their damage. Although our bodies produce their own antioxidants, these often become damaged as we age, so introducing antioxidants into our bodies allows these nutrients and enzymes to assist in chemical reactions which destroy the oxidants or free radicals. The study demonstrates that clove bud essential oil and one of its main components, eugenol, are moderate antioxidants, aiming to detox the body of free radicals that lead to disease.

Reference

http://www.ncbi.nlm.nih.gov/pubmed/22145105

http://www.ncbi.nlm.nih.gov/pmc/articles/PMC3221489/pdf/scipharm-2011-79-779.pdf]

Chapter 4 – The Ins & Outs of Essential Oils

Where do essential oils come from?

Plants and plant species naturally produce essential oils for various reasons, one being to draw pollinator insects to them, another being to repel invading organisms (bacteria, animals). A number of chemical compounds compose each plant's essential oil, and the combination of these compounds are specific to each oil, which then instills in the oil its own unique properties. Essential oils can be harnessed from all sorts of plant components, including flowers, leaves, bark, fruit, roots, and resin. For instance, cinnamon oil is harnessed from bark, lemon oil from the peel, and lavender oil from lavender flowers. Certain plants can produce a few chemical variants of the same essential oil, which are acquired from different parts of the plant.

Some of these parts produce a large amount of oil, while others produce just a smidgen. The oil's quality and potency depends upon a number of factors, including the subspecies of the plant, its soil conditions, the time of year and even the time of day you harvest it.

How are essential oils extracted?

Essential oils can be extracted from plants through various methods, including pressing, distillation, solvent and maceration. Let's take a brief look at each:

Pressing Method

Commonly used with citrus fruit, the pressing method extracts the oil through a technique which involves pushing the fruit peels through a press. Oily fruits and plants are best suited for this technique. Orange oil, for example, is extracted from orange skins through the pressing method.

Distillation Method

This technique harkens back to the days of old-timey moonshiners, as the same sort of method used to create strong liquor can be used to extract essential oils. Using a still, boiled water and plant materials will create steam which is then cooled by coils and condensed into a combination of water and oil. This combination doesn't mix, so the oil can then be extracted from it.

Solvent Method

Through a multi-step process, certain plant and flower

oils can be extracted using alcohol and other solvents, which extort the essential oil from the plant materials.

Maceration Method

When a "carrier" or fixed oil or lard is mixed with the plant material and set out in the sun, over a period of time, the carrier oil is infused with the plant's essence. Heat sources, other than the sun, are often used to speed the process. Throughout the process, more plant material is added to produce a more potent oil.

How do you use essential oils?

Although some studies about the effectiveness of essential oils are conducted by small companies or even individuals, several them are conducted by the food and cosmetic industries. In general, the pharmaceutical industry shows next to no interest in herbal medicine, primarily because there are few options to patent such products. Being as such, the product's lack of profitability results in a lack of research funding. Regardless, the historical uses of essential oils tell us what we need to know: these oils have been effectively administered for centuries. The therapeutic qualifications of essential oils can be plotted in the survival of humanity across cultures and generations.

Another reason that studies on essential oils have not resulted in much conclusive evidence as to their overall effectiveness is because definitive results are sometimes difficult to prove, as the quality of each batch of oil can vary for several reasons. One is that essential oils are impossible to standardize. As mentioned above, even the slightest variance in soil conditions and the time of harvesting – as well as innumerable other factors – will produce a different product quality and potency. In addition, essential oils are often obtained from various species of the same plant; Eucalyptus radiata and Eucalyptus globulus can both be used in the making of therapeutic-grade eucalyptus oil and, as a result, they may have slightly different properties and degrees of strength or effectiveness.

Just as there are several methods by which to extract essential oils, there are several methods to administer them therapeutically. The variety of chemical compounds in each essential oil means that their benefits and applications also vary across the board. Below are a few of these methods.

Topical Administration

Direct application of many essential oils works like a sponge, as skin sops up chemicals and other things (like sunlight, for instance). Topical application is best when you want to clear up an ailment on the skin's surface or in the underlying muscle tissue. When applying topically, you may either massage the oil into the skin or simply dab on the skin for therapeutic results. You might combine the essential oil with a carrier oil for topical use to dilute its potency. This is safer, as the oil is so concentrated. You may support your body's defenses against rash or muscle pain in this manner, but you should always test your patient for allergens before applying. Adverse effects are produced by natural chemicals as much as synthetic ones; poison ivy, for example.

To test for allergens, place a drop or two on your patient's inner forearm. If a rash develops within 12 to 24 hours, then the patient is allergic. In addition, phototoxicity – sun exposure resulting in an exacerbated burn – may be an issue when citrus oils are applied topically. So, one must proceed with caution when applying essential oils using this method.

Inhalation Therapy

Commonly known as "aromatherapy", this essential oil application is effective for inner ailments, like sore throat or cold. In a steaming bowl of distilled or sterilized water, add a few drops of essential oil and, with a towel over your head, bend over the bowl and inhale. The towel captures the vapors, making the technique even more effective. Essential oils can also be placed in a diffuser or potpourri throughout a room to produce somewhat diluted medicinal effects.

Ingestion

When using this method, proceed with caution. Direct ingestion of essential oils must be monitored and applied in small doses that are diluted in a tablespoon or more of any carrier oil – olive oil, for example. If you are unsure of dosage amounts, make a tea with the relevant herb instead. Although the effects of this diluted use may be weaker, this application is a better alternative than an overdose of essential oils.

What are the general benefits of using essential oils?

Replacement for Prescription Drugs

One practical benefit for using essential oils is, of course, their substitutive nature. Many believe that they can replace Rx drugs, which is the ultimate reason to educate yourself on their application and to begin stockpiling your essential oil supply. Although it is our opinion that 100% pure essential oils that carry no harmful side effects are better to support the body and its functions, we recommend that you consult your physician before replacing your prescription or over-the-counter medications.

One of the potential threats of economic or social collapse is the lack of resources, and primarily the inability to procure prescription drugs. Being as such, finding suitable alternatives should be a priority when prepping for the worst.

Their portability is also a major bonus when it comes to survival prepping. The fact that these ultra-concentrated oils take up little-to-no space makes toting them to your shelter all the simpler should the need arise. And, because essential oils are highly concentrated, the application used in most procedures requires only a drop or two of oil, which means that tiny bottle will be long-lasting (example 15mL bottle contains approx. 250 drops).

Cheap, but Effective Alternative

Though money may be the last thing on your mind when it comes to prepping for a survival situation (money may even be obsolete in the event of social collapse), it is worth noting that the expense of essential oils pales in comparison to prescription drugs. In fact, whether you are forced to survive on essential oils due to a lack of prescription reserves, in some cases, you might consider substituting your prescriptions for these inexpensive alternatives regardless. Essential oils are a cheap, but equally effective alternative to prescription medicine.

No Expiration Date

Another benefit of essential oils is that they do not expire, neither do they have "proper storage" requirements. Several medicines and medicinal products must be replaced every couple years, so this sets essential oils ahead of the pack when it comes to shelf life.

Versatility

Essential oils also offer great versatility. Apart from providing wellness benefits, essential oils can be repurposed for household and hygienic applications. For instance, if you're looking for something that might serve your dental hygiene needs in a time of crisis, thieves oil is your go-to essential oil. If you want to maintain your skin's wellness, frankincense and lavender will do the trick; the latter also serves as sunscreen, so you can prevent sun damage as well.

When it comes to the house or shelter, you can use

essential oils to deodorize, which will come in handy in a disaster scenario where things might start to smell fishy due to lack of proper utilities and care. For example, after the 2011 tsunami and the subsequent nuclear reactor meltdown in Japan, a nurse named Risa Nakahira used essential oils to deodorize and sanitize putrid public bathrooms in overpopulated evacuation facilities. As relief workers searched for survivors, often wading through debris and decay, Nakahira also deodorized their boots and masks using essential oils. The possibilities of these natural oils are endless.

They are also versatile when it comes to the range of patients they're capable of supporting. The wellness of everyone from your great grandfather to your infant baby can be fortified with the aid of essential oils in the appropriate dosage. They even come in handy when supporting livestock or pets. From teething infants to dementia in the elderly, from teenagers with acne to dogs with urinary tract infections, essential oils can serve any patient with nearly any ailment.

Conclusion

Now that you know all about what clove bud essential oil can do for you – where it originates, how it's extracted, its benefits and properties, and the different methods of administration – you can use it confidently to support the body's defenses against wellness issues and start to assemble a kit of essential oils for survival. Essential oils can be purchased online or at your local holistic treatment store. If you intend to stock up through online sources, visit: EverythingEssential.com or other like sites.

The various benefits of essential oils and their properties are countless. To build your own kit, first focus on acquiring the essential oils which may bear more relevance to your wellness issues or the potential wellness threats within your environment. When it comes to cold and flu season, for instance, clove bud essential oil will be one of your more crucial oils, due to its immune-supportive properties.

Used as a supplement or as your go-to for stress disorders, skin care, or respiratory issues, the application of clove bud essential oil in medicine has survived for centuries and will survive centuries more. When it comes down to it, you don't need to rely on pharmaceuticals; essential oils, herbs, and plenty of other natural ingredients can be used to help support any number of wellness issues, whether ailment or injury.

Essential oils are essential to your survival in the case of viral outbreak, social collapse or natural disaster because, when the SHTF, your access to pharmaceuticals will likely either be limited or eliminated altogether. Alternatives to our modern-day standard will equate survival when no other option exists. And when it comes to a life-or-death situation, you can't let your wellness decline, no matter the state of the world.

DISCLAIMER AND/OR LEGAL NOTICES: Every effort has been made to accurately represent this book and it's potential. Results vary with every individual, and your results may or may not be different from those depicted. No promises, guarantees or warranties, whether stated or implied, have been made that you will produce any specific result from this book. Your efforts are individual and unique, and may vary from those shown. Your success depends on your efforts, background and motivation.

The material in this publication is provided for educational and informational purposes only and is not intended as medical advice. The information contained in this book should not be used to diagnose or treat any illness, metabolic disorder, disease or health problem. Always consult your physician or healthcare provider before beginning any nutrition or exercise program. Use of the programs, advice, and information contained in this book is at the sole choice and risk of the reader.